The Vibrant Das Colle

Quick and Easy Guide for Begin
Back in Shape

Demi Cooper

Table of contents

Garden Vegetable and Herb Soup

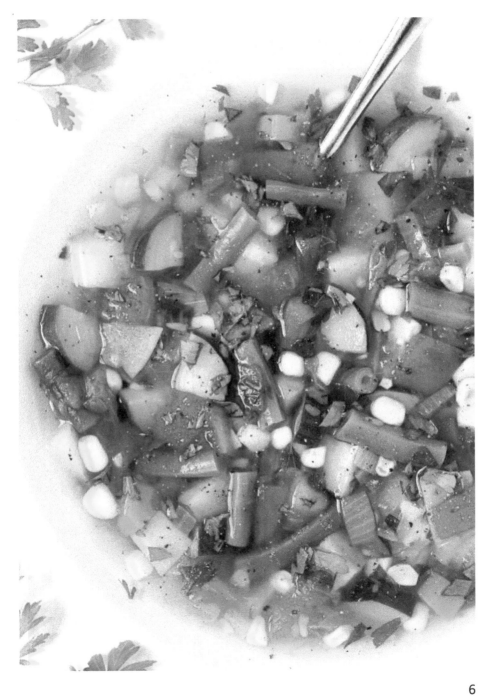

Total Time

Prep: 20 min. Cook: 30 min.

Makes 8 servings (2 quarts)

Ingredients:

- 2 tablespoons olive oil
- 2 medium onions, hacked
- 2 huge carrots, cut
- 1 pound red potatoes (around 3 medium), cubed
- 2 cups of water
- 1 can (14-1/2 ounces) diced tomatoes in sauce
- 1-1/2 cups vegetable soup
- 1-1/2 teaspoons garlic powder
- 1 teaspoon dried basil
- 1/2 teaspoon salt
- 1/2 teaspoon paprika
- 1/4 teaspoon dill weed
- 1/4 teaspoon pepper
- 1 medium yellow summer squash, split and cut
- 1 medium zucchini, split and cut

Directions:

1.   In a huge pan, heat oil over medium warmth. Include onions and carrots; cook and mix until onions are delicate, 4-6 minutes. Include potatoes and cook 2 minutes. Mix in water, tomatoes, juices, and seasonings. Heat to the point of boiling. Diminish heat; stew, revealed, until potatoes and carrots are delicate, 9 minutes.

2.   Include yellow squash and zucchini; cook until vegetables are delicate, 9 minutes longer. Serve or, whenever wanted, puree blend in clusters, including extra stock until wanted consistency is accomplished.

Super-easy Chicken Noodle Soup

SmartPoints value: Green plan - 3SP, Blue plan - 2SP, Purple plan - 2SP

Total Time: 32 min, Prep time: 12 min, Cooking time: 20 min, Serves: 8

Nutritional value: Calories - 351.3, Carbs - 37.3g, Fat - 4.5g, Protein - 39.7g

In this recipe, I will make it easy for you to prepare a hearty soup for the whole family, all with just one pot. A big cup of 1 1/2 portion has only two SmartPoints value, so it's perfect for lunch, either to take to work or for your child's lunchbox, too.

Unlike other recipes like it, this one will be ready in just 32 minutes, not hours!

Now, pick up some ZeroPoint chicken breasts, frozen vegetables, a box of pasta, chicken broth, and a few more bits and pieces, and let's get you started on this family delight.

Ingredients

Black pepper - ¼ tsp

- Chicken breast(s) (cooked) - 6 oz, chopped (skinless, boneless)
- Salted butter - 2 tsp
- Onion(s) (uncooked)- 1 large, well chopped
- Table salt - 1½ tsp, divided
- Chicken broth (reduced-sodium) - 64 oz
- Pasta (uncooked) - 4 oz, small shape such as ditalini (about 1 cup)
- Mixed vegetables (frozen) - 10 oz, such as peas, green beans, and carrots
- Tomatoes (canned) - 15 oz, petite cut, rinsed and drained
- Parmesan cheese (grated) - 1 Tbsp
- Lemon juice (fresh) - 2 tsp
- Fresh chives - ¼ cup(s), chopped (optional)

Instructions

1.   Melt two teaspoons of butter in a large stockpot over medium-low heat.

2.   Add well-chopped onion and 1/2 teaspoon of salt, then cook, often stirring, until the onion is soft and translucent; about 10 minutes.

3.   Add the broth in the chicken and increase the heat to high, then bring it to a boil.

4.   Put in the pasta, frozen vegetables, and tomatoes, then cook until pasta is soft; about 7 minutes.

5.   Stir in the chicken, lemon juice, cheese, remaining one teaspoon of salt, black pepper, and chives, then cook one more minute to heat through.

Hearty Ginger Soup

Serving: 4

Prep Time: 5 minutes

Cook Time: 5 minutes

Ingredients:

- 3 cups coconut almond milk
- 2 cups water
- ½ pound boneless chicken breast halves, cut into chunks
- 3 tablespoons fresh ginger root, minced
- 2 tablespoons fish sauce
- ¼ cup fresh lime juice
- 2 tablespoons green onions, sliced
- 1 tablespoon fresh cilantro, chopped

How To:
1. Take a saucepan and add coconut almond milk and water.
2. Bring the mixture to a boil and add the chicken strips.
3. Reduce the warmth to medium and simmer for 3 minutes.
4. Stir within the ginger, juice , and fish sauce.

5.   Sprinkle a couple of green onions and cilantro.

6.   Serve!

Nutrition (Per Serving)

Calories: 415

Fat: 39g

Carbohydrates: 8g

Protein: 14g

Tasty Tofu and Mushroom Soup

Serving: 8

Prep Time: 10 minutes

Cook Time: 10 minutes

Ingredients:

- 3 cups prepared dashi stock
- ¼ cup shiitake mushrooms, sliced
- 1 tablespoon miso paste
- 1 tablespoon coconut aminos
- 1/8 cup cubed soft tofu
- 1 green onion, diced

How To:

1.   Take a saucepan and add stock, bring back a boil.
2.   Add mushrooms, cook for 4 minutes.
3.   Take a bowl and add coconut aminos, miso paste and blend well.

4.   Pour the mixture into stock and let it cook for six minutes on simmer.

5.   Add diced green onions and enjoy!

Nutrition (Per Serving)

Calories: 100

Fat: 4g

Spring Soup and Poached Egg

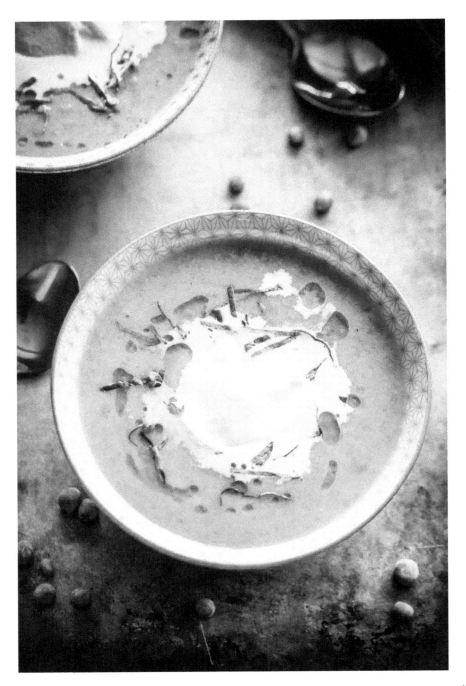

Serving: 4

Prep Time: 5 minutes

Cook Time: 15 minutes

Ingredients:

- 2 whole eggs
- 32 ounces chicken broth
- 1 head romaine lettuce, chopped

How To:

1.   Bring the chicken broth to a boil.

2.   Reduce the heat and poach the 2 eggs in the broth for 5 minutes.

3.   Take two bowls and transfer the eggs into a separate bowl.

4.   Add chopped romaine lettuce into the broth and cook for a few minutes.

5.   Serve the broth with lettuce into the bowls.

6.   Enjoy!

Nutrition (Per Serving)

Calories: 150

Fat: 5g

Carbohydrates: 6g

Protein: 16

Lobster Bisque

Serving: 4

Prep Time: 10 minutes

Cook Time: 15 minutes

Ingredients:

- ¾ pound lobster, cooked and lobster
- 4 cups chicken broth
- 2 garlic cloves, chopped
- ¼ teaspoon pepper
- ½ teaspoon paprika
- 1 yellow onion, chopped
- ½ teaspoon salt
- 14 ½ ounces tomatoes, diced
- 1 tablespoon coconut oil
- 1 cup low fat cream

How To:

1.   Take a stockpot and add the coconut oil over medium heat.

2.   Then sauté the garlic and onion for 3 to 5 minutes.

3.   Add diced tomatoes, spices and chicken broth and bring to a boil.

4.   Reduce to a simmer, then simmer for about 10 minutes.

5.   Add the warmed heavy cream to the soup.

6.   Blend the soup till creamy by using an immersion blender.

7.   Stir in cooked lobster.

8.   Serve and enjoy!

Nutrition (Per Serving)

Calories: 180

Fat: 11g

Carbohydrates: 6g

Protein: 16g

Tomato Bisque

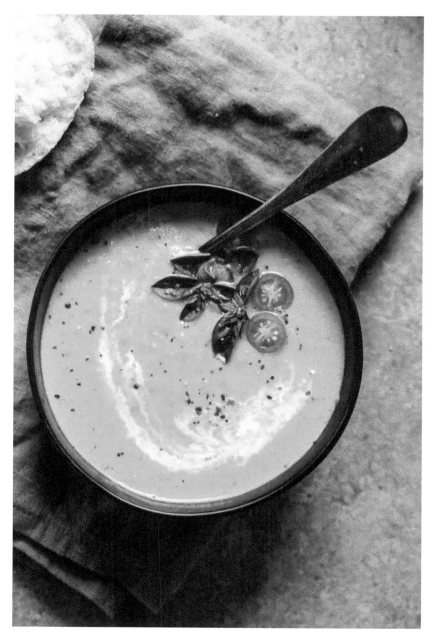

Serving: 4

Prep Time: 10 minutes

Cook Time: 40 minutes

Ingredients:

- 4 cups chicken broth
- 1 cup low fat cream
- 1 teaspoon thyme dried
- 3 cups canned whole, peeled tomatoes
- 2 tablespoons almond butter
- 3 garlic cloves, peeled
- Pepper as needed

How To:

1. Take a stockpot and first add the butter to the bottom of a stockpot.
2. Then add all the ingredients except heavy cream into it.
3. Bring to a boil.
4. Simmer for 40 minutes.
5. Warm the heavy cream and stir into the soup.
6. Serve and enjoy!

Nutrition (Per Serving)

Calories: 141

Fat: 12g

Carbohydrates: 4g

Protein: 4g

Chipotle Chicken Chowder

Serving: 4

Prep Time: 10 minutes

Cook Time: 23 minutes

Ingredients:

- 1 medium onion, chopped
- 2 garlic cloves, minced
- 6 bacon slices, chopped
- 4 cups jicama, cubed
- 3 cups chicken stock
- 1 teaspoon salt
- 2 cups low-fat, cream1 tablespoon olive oil
- 2 tablespoons fresh cilantro, chopped
- 1 ¼ pounds chicken, thigh boneless, cut into 1 inch chunks
- ½ teaspoon pepper
- 1 chipotle pepper, minced

How To:

1.   Heat olive oil over medium heat in a large sized saucepan, add bacon.

2. Cook until crispy, add onion, garlic, and jicama.

3. Cook for 7 minutes, add chicken stock and chicken.

4. Bring to a boil and reduce temperature to low.

5. Simmer for 10 minutes

6. Season with salt and pepper.

7. Add heavy cream and chipotle, simmer for 5 minutes.

8. Sprinkle chopped cilantro and serve, enjoy!

Nutrition (Per Serving)

Calories: 350

Fat: 22g

Carbohydrates: 8g

Protein: 22g

Bay Scallop Chowder

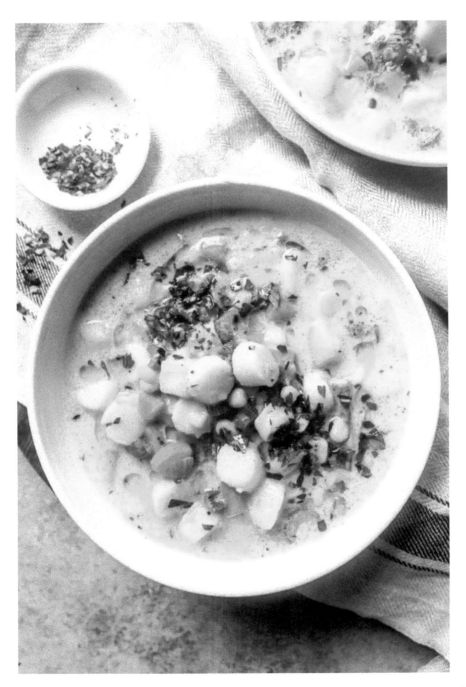

Serving: 4

Prep Time: 10 minutes

Cook Time: 18 minutes

Ingredients:

- 1 medium onion, chopped
- 2 ½ cups chicken stock
- 4 slices bacon, chopped
- 3 cups daikon radish, chopped
- ½ teaspoon dried thyme
- 2 cups low-fat cream
- 1 tablespoon almond butter
- Pepper to taste
- 1 pound bay scallops

How To:

1.   Heat olive over medium heat in a large sized saucepan, add bacon and cook until crisp, add onion and daikon radish.

2.   Cook for 5 minutes, add chicken stock.

3.   Simmer for 8 minutes, season with salt and pepper, thyme.
4. Add heavy cream, bay scallops, simmer for 4 minutes

4.   Serve and enjoy!

Nutrition (Per Serving)

Calories: 307

Fat: 22g

Carbohydrates: 7g

Protein: 22g

Broiled Tilapia

SmartPoints value: Green plan - 2SP, Blue plan - 0SP, Purple plan - 0SP

Total Time: 13 min, Prep time: 8 min, Cooking time: 5 min, Serves: 4

Nutritional value: Cal - 154.8, Carbs - 1.5g, Fat - 6.4g, Protein - 22.8g

You can apply this recipe with other types of fish, such as sole, halibut, flounder, and even shellfish. You also swap lime juice for lemon juice.

Ingredients

- Black pepper - ¼ tsp, freshly ground
- Cooking spray - 1 spray(s)
- Garlic (herb seasoning) - 2 tsp
- Lemon juice (fresh) - 1 Tbsp
- Table salt - ½ tsp (or to taste)
- Tilapia fillet(s) (uncooked) - 20 oz, four 5 oz fillets

Instructions

1.   Prepare your grill by preheating. Coat a skillet with cooking spray.

2.   Apply seasoning to both sides of the fish with salt and pepper.

3.   Transfer the fish to the prepared skillet and drizzle it with lemon juice, then sprinkle garlic herb seasoning over the top.

4.   Broil the fish until it is fork-tender; about 5 minutes.

Grilled Miso-Glazed Cod

SmartPoints value: Green plan - 3SP, Blue plan - 2SP, Purple plan - 2SP

Total Time: 35 min, Prep time: 10 min, Cooking time: 15 min, Serves: 4

Nutritional value: Cal - 227.2, Carbs - 15.0g, Fat - 3.1g, Protein - 30.0g

This marinade produces a fantastic glaze for grilled cod. You can pair it with grilled scallions, drizzled with low-sodium soy sauce, and sesame oil to make a complete meal. If you don't have a fish basket, put foil on one area of your grill to prevent the fish from sticking out below it. Alternatively, you can broil the fish instead. Cod makes a perfect choice for grilling. Flip the fish when it starts to flake and turn opaque. Use a spatula with a broader mouth when turning the fish to help prevent the fish from breaking apart when turning. It is preferable to serve this dish with roasted carrots or broccoli.

Ingredients

- White miso - 3 Tbsp
- Sugar (dark brown) - 1½ Tbsp
- Sake - 1 Tbsp
- Mirin - ½ fl oz, (1 Tbsp)
- Atlantic cod (uncooked) - 20 oz, (fillets, skin removed

- Cooking spray - 1 spray(s)
- Uncooked scallion(s) (chopped) - 2 Tbsp

Instructions

1.   Whisk together miso, sugar, sake, and mirin in a small bowl and spread the mixture over the cod. Cover the cod and refrigerate for at least 2 hours or up to 24 hours.

2.   Coat a grill pan off the heat with cooking spray and preheat to medium heat.

3.   Remove the cod from marinade (reserve marinade). Place it in a fish grilling basket and grill until the cod is opaque and flakes easily with a fork.

4.   Grill each side for about 5 to 7 min (brush the cod with the remaining marinade half-way through the grilling phase to create a thicker glaze). Serve the cod garnished with scallions.

Grilled Tuna with Herb Butter

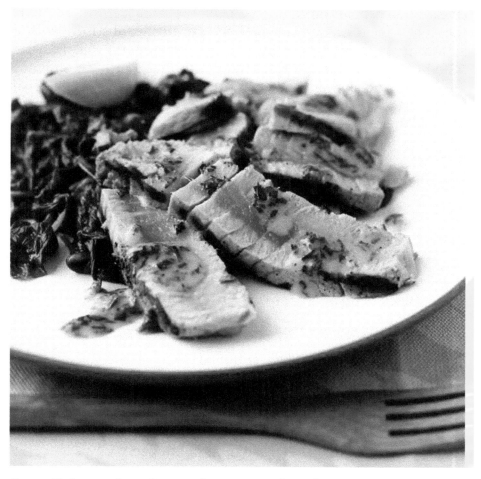

SmartPoints value: Green plan - 4SP, Blue plan - 3SP, Purple plan - 3SP

Total Time: 18 min, Prep time: 12 min, Cooking time: 6 min, Serves: 4

Nutritional value: Calories - 192.0, Carbs - 8.3g, Fat - 2.5g, Protein - 38.3g

You can prepare this grilled tuna recipe in under 20 minutes. Drizzle some olive oil and lime over the tuna before you start cooking it for a unique flavor. You can nicely substitute with a lemon if you don't have a lime. I will recommend that you use salted butter for the sauce instead of unsalted butter to enhance the flavor of the dish. The secret ingredient in this grilled fish recipe is the freshly made herb butter. It also tastes great when drizzled over the spinach.

Ingredients

- Olive oil - 1 tsp
- Lime juice (fresh) - 1 tsp
- Black pepper - ⅛ tsp, or to taste
- Cooking spray - 1 spray(s)
- Salted butter - 2 Tbsp, softened
- Chives (finely chopped) - 1 Tbsp, fresh
- Parsley (fresh) - 1 Tbsp, finely chopped
- Tarragon (fresh) - 1 Tbsp, finely chopped
- Lime zest (fresh, minced) - 1 tsp
- Table salt - ¼ tsp, or to taste
- Spinach (fresh) - 1 pound(s), baby-variety, steamed
- Yellowfin tuna (uncooked) - 1 pound(s), one steak cut 1- to 1-1/2 inches thick

Instructions

1.   Drizzle oil and lime juice on both sides of the fish and set it aside.

2.   Coat your grill with cooking spray off heat, and preheat the grill on high heat.

3.   Combine softened butter, chives, parsley, tarragon, lime zest, salt, and pepper in a small metal bowl and then set aside.

4.   Grill the tuna on one side for three minutes, then carefully turn it and cook on the other side for another three minutes or longer until you have achieved the desired degree of cooking.

5.   Place the bowl containing butter mixture on the grill just until it melts. Don't let it cook.

6.   Slice the tuna thinly and serve it over spinach, then drizzle melted herb butter over the top.

Notes: If you prefer, you can broil the tuna on a grill pan. In this recipe, you will prepare the tuna like a steak. In case you prefer your tuna to be more well done, add about 1 minute to your total cooking time. However, tuna cooks rapidly, so make sure you do not overcook it. The herb butter is excellent on both the tuna and the spinach.

Lemon-Herb Roasted Salmon

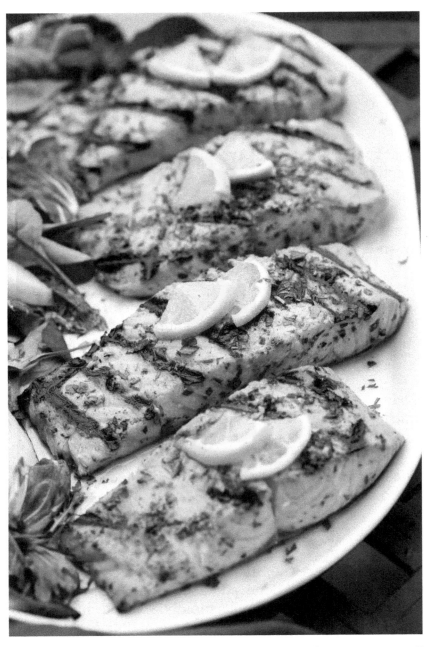

SmartPoints value: Green plan - 5SP, Blue plan - 2SP, Purple plan - 2SP

Total Time: 31 min, Prep time: 16 min, Cooking time: 15 min, Serves: 4

Nutritional value: Calories - 118.1, Carbs - 1.0g, Fat - 6.8g, Protein - 12.9g

Give your family a fabulous salmon flavor with lemon juice, lemon zest, and fresh herbs in this easy entrée that will be ready in about 30 minutes. I have used pink salmon fillets because they are less fatty compared to some other salmon varieties like sockeye and Coho salmon.

The salmon should flake when pierced with a fork. That's an excellent indicator that it is ready. Ensure that you zest the lemon before juicing it.

To produce enough zest and juice for this recipe, you will need about two lemons. The mix of fresh herbs in this dish is lovely. However, you can use whatever combination you like; this recipe is versatile. Stir a few red pepper flakes into the herb mixture to add a little heat.

Ingredients

- Black pepper (coarsely ground) - ⅛ tsp (or to taste)
- Cooking spray - 1 spray(s)
- Lemon juice (fresh) - 4 Tbsp, divided
- Lemon zest (finely grated) - 1 tsp (with extra for garnish, if you like)

- Minced garlic - 1 tsp

- Oregano (fresh) - 1 tsp

- Parsley (fresh, chopped) - 1 Tbsp (with extra for garnish, if you like)

- Uncooked wild pink salmon fillet(s) (also known as humpback salmon) - 1½ pound(s), four 6-oz pieces about 1-inch-thick each

- Table salt - ⅛ tsp (or to taste)

- Sugar - 1½ Tbsp

- Thyme (fresh, chopped) - 1 Tbsp (with extra for garnish, if you like)

Instructions

1.   Heat your oven to 400°F before using it. Get a small, shallow baking dish and coat it with cooking spray.

2.   Apply seasoning to both sides of the salmon with salt and pepper, then place the salmon in the prepared baking dish and drizzle on it with two tablespoons of lemon juice.

3.   Whisk the remaining two tablespoons of lemon juice, sugar, parsley, thyme, lemon zest, garlic, and oregano together in a small bowl, then continue whisking until the sugar dissolves in the mixture and set it aside.

4.   Roast the salmon until it is close to being ready; about 13 minutes, then remove it from the oven and top it with the lemon-herb mixture.

5.   Return it to the oven and allow it to roast until the salmon is fork-tender, about 2 minutes more. Garnish the dish with fresh herbs that you chopped and the grated zest, if you like.

Mango Salsa

SmartPoints value: Green plan - 0SP, Blue plan - 0SP, Purple plan - 0SP

Total time: 15 min, Prep time: 15 min, Cooking time: 0 min, Serves: 4

Nutritional value: Calories – 71, Carbs – 17.7g, Fat – 0.5g, Protein – 1.3g

The mango salsa is a great snack full of fruits and veggies. Although salsa goes well with chips, it doesn't mean that you can use it for other things. However, it's an excellent topper for fish, chicken, and even salads.

Ingredients

- Large mango (peeled and diced) - 1 item
- Red onion (finely chopped) - 1/2
- Red bell pepper (chopped) - 1 cup
- Jalapeno pepper (seeded and chopped) - (1 small piece)
- Garlic (minced) - 2 cloves
- Lime juice - 1 cup
- Pinch of salt (add to taste)

Instructions

1.   Put all the ingredients in a bowl and season as desired with salt.

2.   This mouthwatering sweet and savory salsa awakens your taste buds with delicious flavors. It is fresh, light, and loaded with antioxidants that make it a great pair with tortilla chips.

Watermelon Aguas Frescas

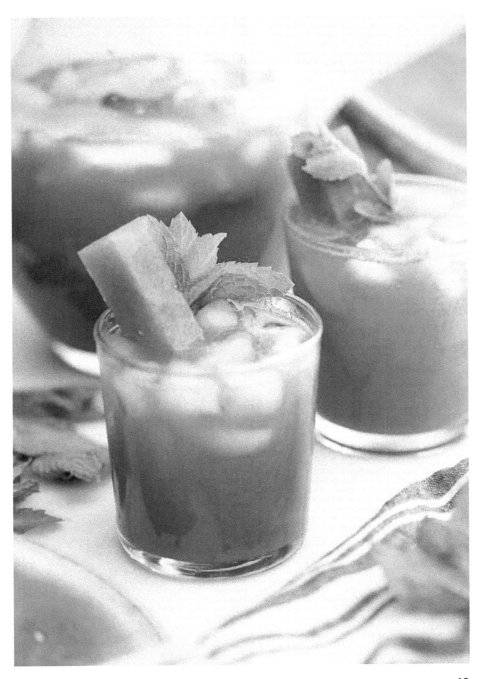

SmartPoints value: 3SP

Total time: 5 min, Prep time: 5 min, Serves - 4

Nutritional value: Calories - 57, Carbs - 14g, Fat - 0g, Protein - 1g

This pure Mexican blend of watermelon, lime juice, water, and a little sugar produces a delightful means of quenching thirst for Weight Watchers on a summer afternoon. You can find an alternative for the cantaloupe if you like.

Ingredients

- Watermelon (seedless, ripe; make sure it's nice and sweet) - 4 cups cubed
- Sugar (honey or agave nectar as an alternative) - 1 tbsp (or to taste)
- Water - 3 cups
- Lime juice (fresh) - 2-3 tsps.
- Mint (fresh) for garnish, if you desire

Instructions

1.   Put the cubed watermelon in a blender and add 1-1/2 cups of the water, the lime juice, and the sugar. Blend everything at high speed until smooth.

2.	Sieve the liquid blend through a medium strainer into a large pitcher (or bowl).

3.	Pour in the remaining 1-1/2 cups of water and stir.

4.	Chill in a refrigerator for 1 hour or longer, depending on the temperature you like.

5.	Drop a few cubes of ice in a glass and pour in the watermelon agua fresca.

6.	Add a mint sprig to garnish if you desire.

Chocolate Peanut Butter Banana Protein Shake

SmartPoints value: 6SP

Total time: 5 min, Prep time: 5 min, Serves: 1

Nutritional value: Calories - 299, Carbs - 29.6g, Fat - 6.1g, Protein - 36.2g

This drink provides a fast, healthy, and delicious way to begin your day, packed with protein to help keep you satisfied until lunchtime.

Ingredients

- Cottage cheese (non-fat) - 1/2 cup
- Peanut Butter Flour (PB2) - 2 tablespoons
- Chocolate protein powder - 1 scoop
- Banana (frozen) - 1/2 finger
- A handful of ice cubes
- Sweetener - to taste (You may not need this if your protein powder already has sweetener in it)

Instructions

1.   Mix all the ingredients in a blender and process until you get a smooth mixture.

2.   You can add more ice cubes to give a thicker consistency to the protein shake.

3.   You can use less ice if you want your drink to be thinner. Add more water.

Skinny Pina Colada

SmartPoints - 7SP

Total time: 5 min, Prep time: 5 min, Serves: 1

Nutritional value: Calories - 183, Carbs - 11g, Fat - 0.5g, Protein - 9.5g

This drink recipe is a cleaned-up version of a pina colada from the Weight Watchers, thickened with vanilla protein powder instead of the cream of coconut. This satisfying and sweet drink has just 7 SmartPoints, which is

about 1/3 of the points of a traditional Pina Colada.

Ingredients

- Vanilla protein powder with about 100 calories per 1-ounce serving (natural) - 3 tablespoons
- Crushed pineapple packed in juice (canned, not drained) - 1/4 cup
- White rum - 1 -1/2 ounces
- Coconut extract - 1/8 teaspoon
- Crushed ice, about eight ice cubes - 1 cup

Instructions

1.   Put all the ingredients in a blender.

2.   Pour in half a cup of water, and blend at high speed until it is smooth.

Spindrift Grapefruit

SmartPoints value: 1SP

Serving size - 355ml

Nutritional value: Calories - 17, Carbs - 4g, Fat - 0g, Protein - 0g

Spindrift is America's first sparkling water fruit drink.

The several varieties of the drink are all created from sparkling water and real squeezed fruits.

Aside from the grapefruit variety, the other types you can enjoy with your meal include blackberry, cucumber, lemon, raspberry lime, orange mango, strawberry, half & half, and cranberry raspberry.

Ingredients

The ingredients of Grapefruit drink include grapefruit juice, lemon juice, orange juice,

Ingenious Eggplant Soup

Serving: 8

Prep Time: 20 minutes

Cook Time: 15 minutes

Ingredients:

- 1 large eggplant, washed and cubed
- 1 tomato, seeded and chopped
- 1 small onion, diced
- 2 tablespoons parsley, chopped
- 2 tablespoons extra virgin olive oil
- 2 tablespoons distilled white vinegar
- ½ cup parmesan cheese, crumbled Sunflower seeds as needed

How To:

1.   Pre-heat your outdoor grill to medium-high.

2.   Pierce the eggplant a couple of times employing a knife/fork.

3. Cook the eggplants on your grill for about quarter-hour until they're charred.

4. forgot and permit them to chill .

5. Remove the skin from the eggplant and dice the pulp.

6. Transfer the pulp to a bowl and add parsley, onion, tomato, olive oil, feta cheese and vinegar.

7. Mix well and chill for 1 hour.

8. Season with sunflower seeds and enjoy!

Nutrition (Per Serving)

Calories: 99

Fat: 7g

Carbohydrates: 7g

Protein:3.4g

Loving Cauliflower Soup

Serving: 6

Prep Time: 10 minutes

Cook Time: 10 minutes

Ingredients:

- 4 cups vegetable stock
- 1-pound cauliflower, trimmed and chopped
- 7 ounces Kite ricotta/cashew cheese
- 4 ounces almond butter
- Sunflower seeds and pepper to taste

How To:

1. Take a skillet and place it over medium heat.

2. Add almond butter and melt.

3. Add cauliflower and sauté for two minutes.

4.   Add stock and convey mix to a boil.

5.   Cook until cauliflower is hard .

6.   Stir in cheese , sunflower seeds and pepper.

7.   Puree the combination using an immersion blender.

8.   Serve and enjoy!

Nutrition (Per Serving)

Calories: 143

Fat: 16g

Carbohydrates: 6g

Protein: 3.4g

Simple Garlic and Lemon Soup

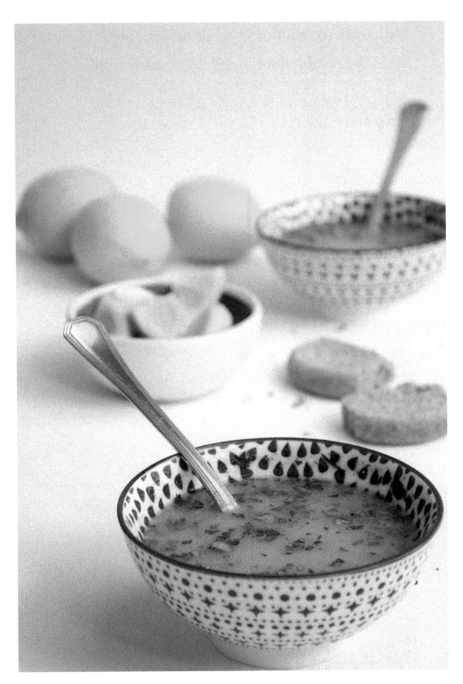

Serving: 3

Prep Time: 10 minutes

Cook Time: nil

Ingredients:

- 1 avocado, pitted and chopped
- 1 cucumber, chopped
- 2 bunches spinach
- 1 ½ cups watermelon, chopped
- 1 bunch cilantro, roughly chopped
- Juice from 2 lemons
- ½ cup coconut amines
- ½ cup lime juice

How To:

1. Add cucumber, avocado to your blender and pulse well.

2. Add cilantro, spinach and watermelon and blend.
3. Add lemon, juice and coconut amino.

4.   Pulse a couple of more times.

5.   Transfer to bowl and enjoy!

Nutrition (Per Serving)

Calories: 100

Fat: 7g

Carbohydrates: 6g

Protein: 3g

Healthy Cucumber Soup

Serving: 4

Prep Time: 14 minutes

Cook Time: Nil

Ingredients:

- 2 tablespoons garlic, minced
- 4 cups English cucumbers, peeled and diced ½ cup onions, diced
- 1 tablespoon lemon juice 1 ½ cups vegetable broth ½ teaspoon sunflower seeds ¼ teaspoon red pepper flakes
- ¼ cup parsley, diced
- ½ cup Greek yogurt, plain

How To:

1.   Add the listed ingredients to a blender and blend to emulsify (keep aside ½ cup of chopped cucumbers).

2.   Blend until smooth.

3.   Divide the soup amongst 4 servings and top with extra cucumbers.

4.   Enjoy chilled!

Nutrition (Per Serving)

Calories: 371

Fat: 36g

Carbohydrates: 8g

Protein: 4g

Salmon and Vegetable Soup

Serving: 4

Prep Time: 10 minutes

Cook Time: 22 minutes

Ingredients:

- 2 tablespoons extra-virgin olive oil
- 1 leek, chopped
- 1 red onion, chopped
- Pepper to taste
- 2 carrots, chopped
- 4 cups low stock vegetable stock
- 4 ounces salmon, skinless and boneless, cubed
- ½ cup coconut cream
- 1 tablespoon dill, chopped

How To:

1.   Take a pan and place it over medium heat, add leek, onion, stir and cook for 7 minutes.

2.   Add pepper, carrots, stock and stir.
3.   Boil for 10 minutes.
4.   Add salmon, cream, dill and stir.
5.   Boil for 5-6 minutes.
6.   Ladle into bowls and serve.
7.   Enjoy!

Nutrition (Per Serving)

Calories: 240

Fat: 4g

Carbohydrates: 7g

Protein: 12g

Garlic Tomato Soup

Serving: 4

Prep Time: 15 minutes

Cook Time: 15 minutes

Ingredients:

- Roma tomatoes, chopped
- 1 cup tomatoes, sundried
- 2 tablespoons coconut oil
- 5 garlic cloves, chopped
- 14 ounces coconut milk
- 1 cup vegetable broth
- Pepper to taste
- Basil, for garnish

How To:

1.   Take a pot, heat oil into it.

2.   Sauté the garlic in it for ½ minute.

3.   Mix in the Roma tomatoes and cook for 8-10 minutes.

4.   Stir occasionally.
5.   Add in the rest of the ingredients, except the basil, and stir well.

6.   Cover the lid and cook for 5 minutes.
7.   Let it cool.
8.   Blend the soup until smooth by using an immersion blender.

9.   Garnish with basil.
10.   Serve and enjoy!

Nutrition (Per Serving)

Calories: 240

Fat: 23g

Carbohydrates: 16g

Protein: 7g

Melon Soup

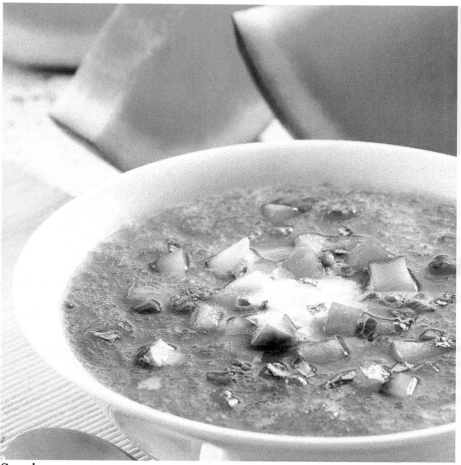

Serving: 4

Prep Time:6 minutes

Cook Time: Nil

Ingredients:

- 4 cups casaba melon, seeded and cubed
- 1 tablespoon fresh ginger, grated

- ¾ cup coconut milk
- Juice of 2 limes

How To:

Add the lime juice, coconut milk, casaba melon, ginger and salt into your blender.

Blend for 1-2 minutes until you get a smooth mixture.

Serve and enjoy!

Nutrition (Per Serving)

Calories: 134

Fat: 9g

Carbohydrates: 13g

Protein: 2g

Spring Salad

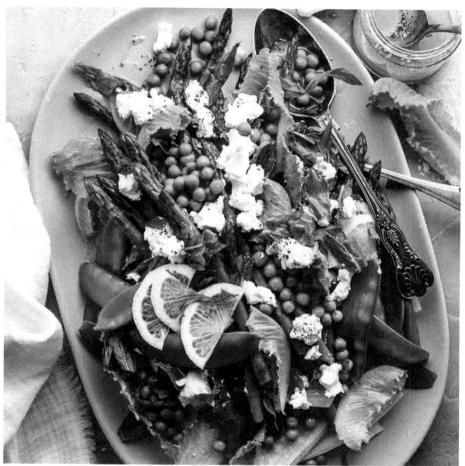

Serving: 2

Prep Time: 10-15 minutes

Cook Time: 0 minutes

Ingredients:

- 2 ounces mixed green vegetables
- 3 tablespoons roasted pine nuts
- 2 tablespoons 5-minute
- 5 Keto Raspberry Vinaigrette

- 2 tablespoons shaved Parmesan
- 2 slices bacon

Pepper as required

How To:

1.   Take a cooking pan and add bacon, cook the bacon until crispy.

2.   Take a bowl and add the salad ingredients and mix well, add crumbled bacon into the salad.
3.   Mix well.
4.   Dress it with your favorite dressing.
5.   Enjoy!

Nutrition (Per Serving)

Calories: 209

Fat: 17g

Net Carbohydrates: 10g

Protein: 4g

Hearty Orange and Onion Salad

Serving: 2

Prep Time: 10 minutes

Cook Time: nil

Ingredients:

6 large oranges

- 3 tablespoons red wine vinegar
- 6 tablespoons olive oil
- 1 teaspoon dried oregano
- 1 red onion, thinly sliced
- 1 cup olive oil
- ¼ cup fresh chives, chopped
- Ground black pepper

How To:

1. Peel orange and cut into 4-5 crosswise slices.

2. Transfer orange to shallow dish.
3. Drizzle vinegar, olive oil on top.
4. Sprinkle oregano.
5. Toss well to mix.
6. Chill for 30 minutes and arrange sliced onion and black olives on top.
7. Sprinkle more chives and pepper.
8. Serve and enjoy!

Nutrition (Per Serving)

Calories: 120

Fat: 6g

Carbohydrates: 20g

Protein: 2g

Grilled Tuna Provencal

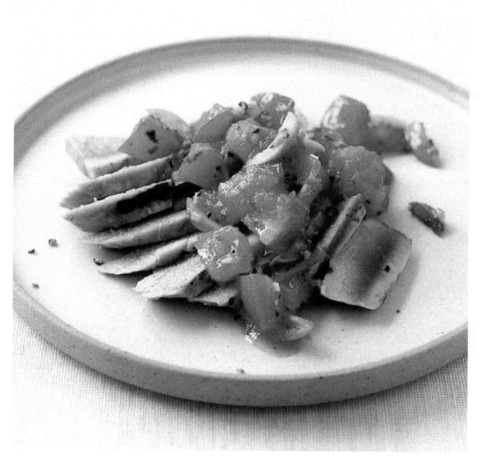

SmartPoints value: Green plan - 3SP, Blue plan - 2SP, Purple plan - 2SP

Total Time: 20 min, Prep time: 10 min, Cooking time: 10 min, Serves: 4

Nutritional value: Calories - 335, Carbs - 14.6g, Fat - 15.5g, Protein - 36.1g

This one-dish meal is usually ready in just 20 minutes, oozing with a delicious French flavor. You can make the whole meal in one pan, aiding clean up after cooking. To cook with a grill pan and get the best result, you need to preheat the pan for at least five minutes to ensure that you distribute the heat evenly. That will help you avoid overcooking parts of the meat while not cooking other parts. If you're not sure about the hotness of the grill pan, drop a half teaspoon of water on there to see if it evaporates.

With steamed spinach or a bed of rice, this dish tastes lovely.

Ingredients

- Black pepper (freshly ground, divided) - ¾ tsp
- Cooking spray - 3 spray(s)
- Uncooked tuna (about 1- to 1 1/2-in thick) - 1 pound(s)
- Olive(s) (pitted and chopped)- 6 large
- Olive oil - 1 Tbsp
- Rosemary (fresh, minced) - 1 Tbsp
- Red wine - 2 fl oz
- Sea salt - ¾ tsp, divided
- Tomato(es) (fresh, diced) - 2½ cup(s)
- Garlic clove(s) (minced) - 2 medium clove(s)
- Parsley (fresh, minced) - 2 Tbsp

- Sugar - ⅛ tsp

Instructions

1.   Wash the tuna thoroughly and pat it dry. Rub 1/4 teaspoon each of salt and pepper over it, then set it aside.

2.   Combine tomatoes, parsley, rosemary, garlic, olives, oil, and the remaining 1/2 teaspoon each of salt and pepper in a separate bowl,

then set it aside.

3.   Get a reasonably large grill pan and coat it with cooking spray, then set it over medium-high heat. When the pan is visibly hot, cook the tuna for 2 to 3 minutes (or longer) per side for a rare cook (or thorough cook). As soon as you have prepared the tuna, remove it to a serving plate and wrap it with aluminum foil to keep it warm.

4.   Add the red wine, tomato mixture, and sugar to the hot grill pan and cook, scraping the bottom of the pan frequently, until the tomato mixture reduces to about two cups. The alcohol must have cooked off.

5.   Remove foil from the tuna, slice it thinly, and serve with tomato mixture over the top.

Grilled Cod Fillets with Lemon Dill Butter

SmartPoints value: Green plan - 3SP, Blue plan - 2SP, Purple plan - 2SP

Total Time: 25 min, Prep time: 15 min, Cooking time: 10 min, Serves: 4

Nutritional value: Calories - 318.7g, Carbs - 6.7g, Fat - 13.0g, Protein - 41.7g

Grill the fish on slices of lemon topped with dill to add a delicious flavor to this dish. Become confident at grilling fish. With the layer of lemon slices, you can easily prevent the fish from sticking to the grate. To make use of a stovetop, prepare a grill pan by preheating it over medium-high heat until it is almost smoking, then continue with the recipe. The mixture of lemon, butter, and dill creates a robust sauce that becomes ready in minutes, even though it tastes like you spent hours preparing it. It is preferable to serve this dish with grilled asparagus.

Ingredients

- Olive oil -2 tsp
- Uncooked Atlantic cod - 24 oz, or another firm white fish like
- tilapia (four 6-oz fillets)
- Table salt - ½ tsp
- Lemon(s) (sliced 1/4-in thick) - 2 medium (you'll need 12 slices total)

- Dill - 2 tsp, chopped
- Dill - 4 sprig(s)
- Light butter - 4 tsp (at room temp.)
- Lemon zest - 1 tsp

Instructions

1.   Get your grill ready by preheating to medium-high heat. Continue the heating for at least 10 minutes after it reaches the desired temperature, then scrape the grate clean with a steel brush and coat it lightly with oil.

2.   While the grill heats up, pat the fish dry and sprinkle salt on it.

3.   Place three lemon slices on the grill carefully, overlapping slightly, and top it with a dill sprig and fish fillet.

4.   Repeat the same with the remaining lemon, dill, and fish. Cover the grill and cook without turning for 8-10 minutes until the fish is opaque all the way through and yields easily to a thin-bladed knife.

5.   While the cooking is on-going, mix the butter, chopped dill, and zest in a small shallow bowl.

6.   Transfer each lemon-dill-fish portion to a plate using two thin-bladed spatulas and top them with 1 1/2 tsp of lemon-dill butter and serve (serving the lemon slices is optional).

Spicy Baked Shrimp

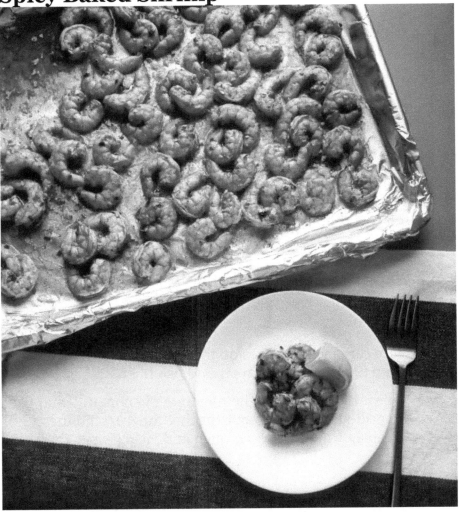

Serving: 4

Prep Time: 10 minutes

Cook Time: 25 minutes + 2-4 hours

Ingredients:

- ½ ounce large shrimp, peeled and deveined
- Cooking spray as needed
- 1 teaspoon low sodium coconut amines
- 1 teaspoon parsley
- ½ teaspoon olive oil
- ½ tablespoon honey
- 1 tablespoon lemon juice

How To:

1. Pre-heat your oven to 450 degrees F.

2. Take a baking dish and grease it well.

3. Mix altogether the ingredients and toss.

4. Transfer to oven and bake for 8 minutes until shrimp turns pink.

5. Serve and enjoy!

Nutrition (Per Serving)

Calories: 321

Fat: 9g

Carbohydrates: 44g

Protein: 22g

Shrimp and Cilantro Meal

Serving: 4

Prep Time: 10 minutes

Cook Time: 5 minutes

Ingredients:

- ¾ pounds shrimp, deveined and peeled
- tablespoons fresh lime juice
- ¼ teaspoon cloves, minced
- ½ teaspoon ground cumin
- 1 tablespoon olive oil
- 1 ¼ cups fresh cilantro, chopped
- 1 teaspoon lime zest
- ½ teaspoon sunflower seeds
- ¼ teaspoon pepper

Direction

1.   Take an outsized sized bowl and add shrimp, cumin, garlic, juice , ginger and toss well.

2.   Take an outsized sized non-stick skillet and add oil, allow the oil to heat up over medium-high heat.

3.   Add shrimp mixture and sauté for 4 minutes.

4.   Remove the warmth and add cilantro, lime zest, sunflower seeds, and pepper.

5.   Mix well and serve hot!

Nutrition (Per Serving)

Calories: 177

Fat: 6g

Carbohydrates: 2g

Protein: 27g

Scallop and Strawberry Mix

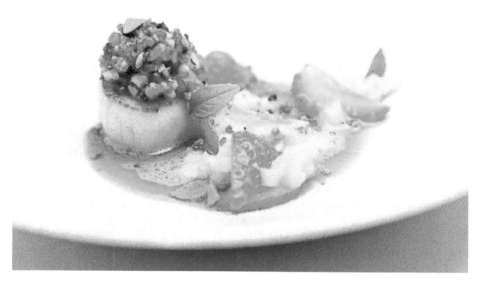

Serving: 4

Prep Time: 10 minutes

Cook Time: 6 minutes

Ingredients:

- ounces scallops
- ½ cup Pico De Gallo
- ½ cup strawberries, chopped

- 1 tablespoon lime juice

Pepper to taste

How To:

1. Take a pan and place it over medium heat, add scallops and cook for 3 minutes on each side .

2. Remove heat.

3. Take a bowl and add strawberries, juice , Pico De Gallo, scallops, pepper and toss well.

4. Serve and enjoy!

Nutrition (Per Serving)

Calories: 169

Fat: 2g

Carbohydrates: 8g

Protein: 13g

Salmon and Orange Dish

Serving: 4

Prep Time: 10 minute

Cook Time: 15 minutes

Ingredients:

- salmon fillets
- cup orange juice
- tablespoons arrowroot and water mixture
- 1 teaspoon orange peel, grated 1 teaspoon black pepper

How To:

1. Add the listed ingredients to your pot.
2. Lock the lid and cook on high for 12 minutes.
3. Release the pressure naturally.
4. Serve and enjoy!

Nutrition (Per Serving)

Calories:583

Fat: 20g

Carbohydrates: 71g

Protein: 33g

Mesmerizing Coconut Haddock

Serving: 3

Prep Time: 10 minutes

Cook Time: 12 minutes

Ingredients:

- Haddock fillets, 5 ounces each, boneless 2 tablespoons coconut oil, melted
- 1 cup coconut, shredded and unsweetened
- ¼ cup hazelnuts, ground Sunflower seeds to taste

How To:

1. Pre-heat your oven to 400 degrees F.
2. Line a baking sheet with parchment paper.
3. Keep it on the side.
4. Pat fish fillets with towel and season with sunflower seeds.
5. Take a bowl and stir in hazelnuts and shredded coconut.
6. Drag fish fillets through the coconut mix until each side are coated well.

7.   Transfer to baking dish.

8.   Brush with copra oil .

9.   Bake for about 12 minutes until flaky.

10.   Serve and enjoy!

Nutrition (Per Serving)

Calories: 299

Fat: 24g

Carbohydrates: 1g

Protein: 20g

Asparagus and Lemon Salmon Dish

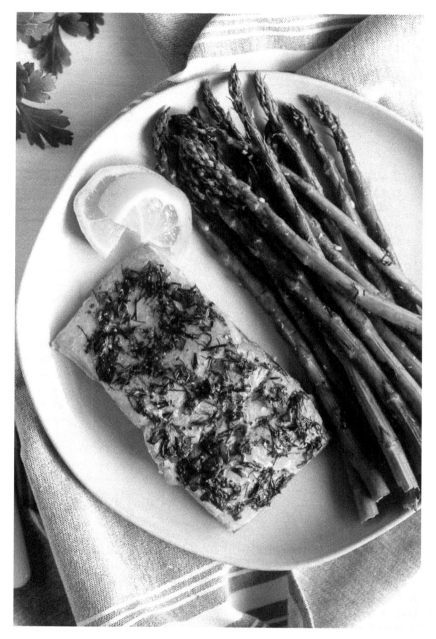

Serving: 3

Prep Time: 5 minutes

Cook Time: 15 minutes

Ingredients:

- 2 salmon fillets, 6 ounces each, skin on Sunflower seeds to taste
- 1-pound asparagus, trimmed 2 cloves garlic, minced tablespoons almond butter ¼ cup cashew cheese

How To:

Pre-heat your oven to 400 degrees F.

Line a baking sheet with oil.

Take a kitchen towel and pat your salmon dry, season as needed.

1.   Put salmon onto the baking sheet and arrange asparagus around it.

2.   Place a pan over medium heat and melt almond butter.

3.   Add garlic and cook for 3 minutes until garlic browns slightly.

4.   Drizzle sauce over salmon.

5.   Sprinkle salmon with cheese and bake for 12 minutes until salmon looks cooked all the way and is flaky.

6.   Serve and enjoy!

Nutrition (Per Serving)

Calories: 434

Fat: 26g

Carbohydrates: 6g

Protein: 42g

Ecstatic "Foiled" Fish

Serving: 4

Prep Time: 20 minutes

Cook Time: 40 minutes

Ingredients:

- 2 rainbow trout fillets
- tablespoon olive oil
- teaspoon garlic salt
- 1 teaspoon ground black pepper
- 1 fresh jalapeno pepper, sliced
- 1 lemon, sliced

How To:

1. Pre-heat your oven to 400 degrees F.
2. Rinse your fish and pat them dry.
3. Rub the fillets with olive oil, season with some garlic salt and black pepper.
4. Place each of your seasoned fillets on a large sized sheet of aluminum foil.

5. Top it with some jalapeno slices and squeeze the juice from your lemons over your fish.

6. Arrange the lemon slices on top of your fillets.

7. Carefully seal up the edges of your foil and form a nice enclosed packet.

8. Place your packets on your baking sheet.

9. Bake them for about 20 minutes.

10. Once the flakes start to flake off with a fork, the fish is ready!

Nutrition (Per Serving)

Calories: 213

Fat: 10g

Carbohydrates: 8g

Protein: 24g

Popcorn

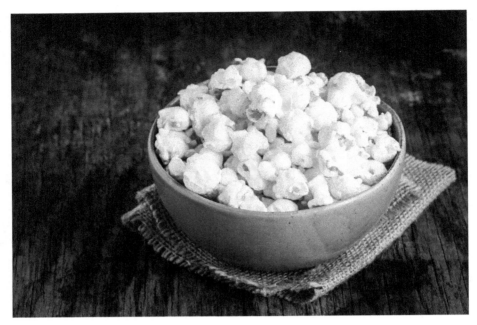

It's a tasty, rather low-calorie snack that can be ready to eat in under 10 minutes. It's perfect if you're craving something a little salty.

Nutritional Facts

servings per container   5

Prep Total   10 min

Serving Size 8

Amount per serving 0%
Calories

      % Daily Value

Total Fat 3g 20%

Saturated Fat 4g   32%

Trans Fat 2g 2%

Cholesterol   2%

Sodium 110mg   0.2%

Total Carbohydrate 21g   50%

Dietary Fiber 9g   1%

Total Sugar 1g   1%

Protein 1g

Vitamin C 7mcg   17%

Calcium 60mg   1%

Iron 7mg   10%

Potassium 23mg   21%

Ingredient & Process

1. Place 2 tablespoons of olive oil and ¼ Cup popcorn in a large saucepan.

2. Cover with a lid, and cook the popcorn over a medium flame, ensuring that you are shaking constantly. Just when you think that it's not working, keep on enduring for another minute or two, and the popping will begin.

3. When the popping stops, take off from the heat and place in a large bowl.

4. Add plenty of salt to taste, and if desired, dribble in ¼ Cup to ½ Cup of melted coconut oil. If you are craving sweet popcorn, add some maple syrup to the coconut oil, about ½ Cup, or to taste.

5 Minutes or Less Vegan Snacks

Here's a list of basically 'no-preparation required' vegan snack ideas that you can munch on anytime:

Nutritional Facts

servings per container   5

Prep Total   10 min

Serving Size   8

Amount per serving 0%
Calories

        % Daily Value

Total Fat 20g   190%

Saturated Fat 2g   32%

Trans Fat 1g 2%

Cholesterol   2%

Sodium 70mg   0.2%

Total Carbohydrate 32g   150%

Dietary Fiber 8g   1%

Total Sugar 1g   1%

Protein 3g

Vitamin C 7mcg   17%

Calcium 210mg   1%

Iron 4mg   10%

Potassium 25mg   20%

Ingredients and Process

1. Trail mix: nuts, dried fruit, and vegan chocolate pieces.

2. Fruit pieces with almond butter, peanut butter or vegan chocolate spread

3. Frozen vegan cake, muffin, brownie or slice that you made on the weekend

4. Vegetable sticks (carrots, celery, and cucumber etc.) with a Vegan Dip (homemade or store-bought) such as hummus or beetroot dip. (Careful of the store-bought ingredients though).

5. Smoothie - throw into the blender anything you can find (within limits!) such as soy milk, coconut milk, rice milk, almond milk, soy yogurt, coconut milk yogurt, cinnamon, spices, sea salt, berries, bananas, cacao powder, vegan

chocolate, agave nectar, maple syrup, chia seeds, flax seeds, nuts, raisins, sultanas... What you put into your smoothie is up to you, and you can throw it all together in less than 5 minutes!

6. Crackers with avocado, soy butter, and tomato slices, or hummus spread.

7. Packet chips (don't eat them too often). There are many vegan chip companies that make kale chips, corn chips, potato chips, and vegetable chips, so enjoy a small bowl now and again.

Fresh Fruit

The health benefits of eating fresh fruit daily should not be minimized. So, make sure that you enjoy some in-season fruit as one of your daily vegan snacks.

Nutritional Facts

servings per container   10

Prep Total   10 min

Serving Size 5/5

Amount per serving 1%
Calories

       % Daily Value

Total Fat 24g 2%

Saturated Fat 8g   3%

Trans Fat 4g 2%

Cholesterol   2%

Sodium 10mg   22%

Total Carbohydrate 7g   54%

Dietary Fiber 4g   1%

Total Sugar 1g   1%

Protein 1g   24

Vitamin C 2mcg   17%

Calcium 270mg   15%

Iron 17mg   20%

Potassium 130mg   2%

Ingredients:

1. Chop your favorite fruit and make a fast and easy fruit salad, adding some squeezed orange juice to make a nice juicy dressing.

2. Serve with some soy or coconut milk yogurt or vegan ice-cream if desired, and top with some tasty walnuts or toasted slithered almonds to make it a sustaining snack.

Vegan Brownie

Nutritional Facts

servings per container   3

Prep Total   10 min

Serving Size 7

Amount per serving 20%
Calories

           % Daily Value

Total Fat 3g   22%

Saturated Fat 22g   8%

Trans Fat 17g   21%

Cholesterol   20%

Sodium 120mg   70%

Total Carbohydrate 30g   57%

Dietary Fiber 4g   8%

Total Sugar 10g   8%

Protein 6g

Vitamin C 1mcg   1%

Calcium 20mg   31%

Iron 2mg   12%

Potassium 140mg   92%

Ingredients:

- 1/2 cup non-dairy butter melted
- 5 tablespoons cocoa
- 1 cup granulated sugar
- 3 teaspoons Ener-G egg replacer
- 1/4 cup water
- 1 teaspoon vanilla
- 3/4 cup flour
- 1 teaspoon baking powder
- 1/2 teaspoon salt
- 1/2 cup walnuts (optional)

Instructions:

1.   Heat oven to 350°. Prepare an 8" x 8" baking pan with butter or canola oil.

2.   Combine butter, cocoa, and sugar in a large bowl.

3.   Mix the egg replacer and water in a blender until frothy.

4.   Add to the butter mixture with vanilla. Add the flour, baking powder, and salt, and mix thoroughly.

5.   Add the walnuts if desired. Pour the batter into the pan, and spread evenly.

6.   Bake for 40 to 45 minutes, or until a toothpick inserted comes out clean.

Italian Chicken Soup with Vegetables

SmartPoints value: Green plan - 4SP, Blue plan - 1SP, Purple plan - 1SP

Total Time: 27 min, Prep time: 15 min, Cooking time: 12 min, Serves: 1

Nutritional value:

Calories - 136.7, Carbs - 22.3g, Fat - 1.0g, Protein - 9.6g

This chicken soup is ideal for a leisurely lunch or a quick dinner, as it is brothy and filled with vegetables. To make it bulky, you can add in any cooked grain you have on hand, like rice, barley, or quinoa, which will also add some nice texture and make it more chewable. You can use any leftover chicken you have. The drizzle of extra virgin olive oil at the end not only makes the soup look a little fancier, but it can also add a rich flavor that takes a simple soup like this one to the next level.

Ingredients

- Chicken broth - 1 cup(s), canned
- Chicken breast(s) - 1 cup(s), diced (skinless, boneless)
- Extra virgin olive oil - 1 tsp, divided
- Fresh thyme - 1¼ tsp (leaves)
- Fresh mushroom(s) - 1 cup(s), sliced
- Garlic clove(s) - 1 medium-sized, minced
- Green beans - 1 small bowl, cooked
- Lemon(s) - 1 slice(s)
- Plum tomato(es) - 1 medium-sized, diced

- Uncooked cauliflower - 1 cup(s), small florets

Instructions

1.   Heat 1/2 tsp of olive oil in a small skillet over medium heat.

2.   Add the mushrooms and garlic, then cook, continuously stirring until mushrooms begin to soften and the mixture is fragrant; about 2 minutes.

3.   Add the broth in the chicken and bring it to a boil over medium-high heat.

4.   Add cauliflower and (or) green beans, then reduce the heat to medium-low and simmer until it is almost tender; about 4 minutes.

5.   Add the chicken, thyme, and tomatoes, then simmer until the vegetables are tender; about 2 minutes.

6.   Drizzle it with the remaining 1/2 tsp of oil and fresh lemon juice, then grind the pepper over the top, if you desire.

Note: You can also garnish your dish with shredded Parmesan cheese (this could add SmartPoints values).

Roasted Chicken Breast with Spiced Cauliflower

SmartPoints value: Green plan - 4SP, Blue plan - 2SP, Purple plan - 2SP

Total Time: 50 min, Prep time: 20 min, Cooking time: 30 min, Serves: 4

Nutritional value: Calories - 470.9, Carbs - 3.5g, Fat - 11.3g, Protein - 84.2g

In this tasty recipe, you will brush chicken breasts with olive oil, turmeric, ground coriander, and cumin, with a touch of cayenne pepper before roasting, and surround it by a bed of cauliflower florets.

After cooking the chicken thoroughly, toss the cauliflower in all the delicious juices in the skillet, and let it continue to roast until it's sweet and tender. You can't have anything more convenient than a single-sheet pan dinner on a busy weeknight.

Drizzle fresh lime juice and sprinkle fresh cilantro into this Indian-influenced

meal to add incredible flavor. In case you don't like cilantro, parsley or oregano works well too.

Ingredients

- Black pepper (divided) - ½ tsp
- Cayenne pepper - ⅛ tsp
- Cooking spray - 2 spray(s)
- Cilantro (finely chopped) - 1 Tbsp
- Olive oil - 2 Tbsp

- Coriander (ground) - 1 tsp

- Turmeric (ground) - 1 tsp

- Durkee Cumin (ground) - ½ tsp

- Kosher salt (divided) - ¾ tsp

- Uncooked chicken breast - 1 pound(s), two 8 oz pieces (boneless, skinless)

- Uncooked cauliflower - 1 pound(s), cut into bite-size pieces

- Fresh lime(s) - ½ medium, with wedges for serving

Instructions

1.   Before you start, heat the oven to 450°F. Get a large baking sheet and line it with parchment paper.

2.   Combine and mix oil, turmeric, coriander, cumin, 1/2 tsp of salt, 1/4 tsp of pepper, and cayenne in a large bowl.
3.   Place the chicken in the center of the prepared baking sheet and brush each piece with 1/2 tsp of oil mixture.

4.   Add cauliflower to the bowl and toss it to coat. Place the cauliflower around the chicken and lightly coat both chicken and cauliflower with cooking spray.

5.   Sprinkle the chicken with the remaining 1/4 tsp of each salt and pepper.

6.   Roast the coated chicken until it cooks through; 15-20 minutes and

let it rest.

7.   Toss the cauliflower and chicken juices in the pan, then continue roasting until browned and tender; about 10 minutes more.

8.   Add the cilantro and toss again.

9.   Thickly slice the chicken across the grain and fan over serving plates.

10.   Serve the cauliflower and chicken in each plate and squeeze 1/2 lime over the top, then serve with additional lime wedges.

Vietnamese Chicken and Veggie Bowl with Rice Noodles

SmartPoints value: Green plan - 6SP, Blue plan - 4SP, Purple plan - 4SP

Total Time: 26 min, Prep time: 20 min, Cooking time: 6 min, Serves: 1

Nutritional value: Calories - 280.4, Carbs - 42.3g, Fat - 10.0g, Protein - 9.1g

This dish is a delicious and stunning entrée that comes together in just 25 minutes. It is a perfect recipe for one. You can even use leftover cooked chicken breast and grilled vegetables.

I would prefer you to use chicken cutlets with broccoli and red peppers, but feel free to experiment with chicken thighs, spinach, mushrooms, onions, or whatever you have on hand.

The soy and fish sauces add that ultimate umami bomb, while sriracha helps keep it balanced out by providing a touch of heat.

You can quickly scale up this recipe if you need to serve it to a crowd. Ingredients

- Cilantro (chopped, fresh leaves) - 2 Tbsp

- Cooked rice noodles - ½ cup(s)

- Asian fish sauce - ½ tsp

- Cooking spray - 4 spray(s)

- Uncooked chicken breast - 5 oz, thin cutlet (boneless, skinless)

- Uncooked broccoli - 1 cup(s), small florets or baby stalks

- Red pepper(s) (sweet) - ½ medium, cut in 2 even pieces

- Soy sauce (low sodium) - 2 Tbsp, divided (or to taste)

- Sriracha sauce - 1 tsp (or to taste)

- Sugar - ¼ tsp

- Roasted peanuts (unsalted dry) - 2 tsp, chopped

Instructions

1.   Coat a grill or grill pan with cooking spray and preheat on medium-high heat.

2.   Place the chicken, broccoli, and red pepper in a shallow bowl and drizzle with one tablespoon of soy sauce, then toss to coat.

3.   Coat the chicken with cooking spray and grill, turning the chicken once and the vegetables a few times, until chicken cooks through and veggies are tender-crisp; about 6 minutes.

4.   Slice the chicken and pepper them into strips, then place all in a bowl over noodles.

5.   Stir together the remaining one tablespoon of soy sauce, fish sauce, and sugar. Drizzle the mixture over your cooked chicken.
6.   Sprinkle a mixture of cilantro, peanuts, and sriracha on the chicken, then serve.

Chicken Tortilla Soup

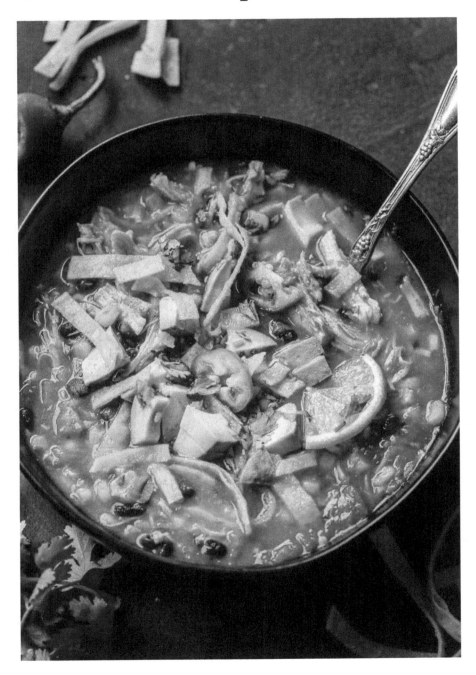

SmartPoints value: Green plan - 4SP, Blue plan - 2SP, Purple plan - 2SP

Total Time: 45 min, Prep time: 15 min, Cooking time: 30 min, Serves: 6

Nutritional value:

Calories - 200, Carbs - 24g, Fat - 9g, Protein - 7g

Preparing this soup is very easy. Once you have chopped and sautéed the vegetables, the rest of the cooking is practically hands-off. You will simmer the chicken in a flavored broth made with fire-roasted tomatoes and lime juice. Doing this will give you some extra minutes to put together a quick

salad or other simple side dishes. Chicken breasts (boneless, skinless) work well in this soup, but you can use chicken thighs as well. If you'd like to make things more interesting, don't de-seed the jalapeño completely.

Ingredients

- Cilantro (chopped) - 1 cup(s)

- Chili powder - 1 tsp

- Chicken broth (reduced-sodium) - 6 cup(s)

- Olive oil - 1 tsp

- Uncooked onion(s) (chopped) - 1½ cup(s)

- Kosher salt -1½ tsp

- Minced Garlic - 4 tsp

- Jalapeño pepper(s) - 1 medium (seeded and minced)

- Tomatoes (canned, diced)- 15 oz, fire roasted-variety, drained

- Uncooked chicken breast - 20 oz (boneless, skinless)
- Lime juice (fresh) - ⅓ cup(s)
- Mexican-style cheese (Shredded reduced) - 6 Tbsp
- Tortilla chips (crushed) - 12 chip(s)

Instructions

1. Set a soup pot over medium heat and preheat.

2. Toss in the chopped onion and salt, then cook, often stirring, until the onion gets soft; 5-10 minutes.

3. Add garlic, chili powder, and jalapeno, then cook for one minute.

4. Put in your broth, tomatoes, lime juice, and chicken, then stir to combine.

5. Simmer and cook until the chicken breasts cook through; about 20 minutes.

6. Remove the chicken breasts from the soup and shred them with two forks, then return the shredded chicken to the pot with cilantro.

7. Serve your soup garnished with tortilla chips and cheese.

Lightning Source UK Ltd.
Milton Keynes UK
UKHW020705130521
383649UK00005B/84